Simply Homeopathy

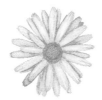

HealthWorks

What is Homeopathy?
A Beginner's Guide

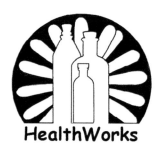

HealthWorks

Simply Homeopathy

What is Homeopathy?
A Beginner's Guide

an introduction to the history,
principles and philosophy
of homeopathy

Jean Osborne LCH, MGH, MHMA
Meryl Hool LCH, MGH, MHMA

Published by
HealthWorks
Osborne Hool Enterprises Limited

First edition 2000

Technology and New Media - James Osborne

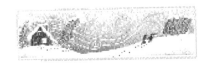

Copyright© illustration Cathy Hill

HealthWorks

Copyright© illustration Joe Revill

A catalogue record for this book is available from the British Library.

Printed by **HealthWorks**

ISBN 0-9538884-1-X

Published by **HealthWorks**
20 Ashford Drive
Kingswood,
Maidstone,
Kent ME17 3PB

HealthWorks is a trading name of Osborne Hool Enterprises Ltd. Registered office: 27 Henley Meadows, Tenterden, Kent TN30 6EN. Registered in England No. 3852487. Directors: Jean Osborne, LCH, MGH, MHMA, and Meryl Hool, LCH, MGH, MHMA.

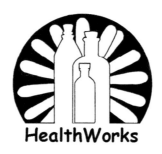

HealthWorks

HealthWorks is a new company formed by professional qualified Homeopaths committed to the introduction of homeopathy to every household. Our practical and easy to follow format will enable you to find the information you need at a glance.

The HealthWorks Objectives

Explain

* and demystify homeopathy
* how to match symptoms with remedies
* how to apply this knowledge safely and effectively

Encourage

* people to take responsibility for their own health
* the accessibility of homeopathy to all
* the application of homeopathy in the home

Enjoy

* confident prescribing for yourself and your family
* the promotion of vitality and well being
* a sense of achievement in your new found knowledge

If you would like to comment on this publication, or have ideas or requests for future literature, please write to us at HealthWorks at the address shown on page 6.

IMPORTANT NOTE

HealthWorks publications have been created as informative literature intended to encourage the safe and effective understanding and use of standard homeopathic remedies in the home on a therapeutic basis.

Homeopathic treating and prescribing is meticulous work. Our aim is to give you an insight into the uniqueness of the individual and the wealth and depth of the philosophy employed within this system of medicine.

Please do not undertake self-treatment of serious or chronic health problems. For this you are recommended to seek the advice of a qualified homeopath or health professional. See page 67.

--ooOoo--

What is Homeopathy?
A Beginner's Guide

CONTENTS PAGE

 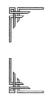
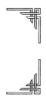

The
History
and
Philosophy
of Homeopathy

an introduction

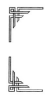 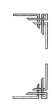

The
History and Philosophy
of Homeopathy

Homeopathic medicine provides a gentle, safe and effective method of treatment for everything from minor ailments to chronic illness.

This introductory book sets out to clarify all your questions about this fascinating subject. As well as providing you with information about the origins and development of homeopathy, we explain in an easy to understand style, how remedies are prepared and what is meant by 'like cures like', 'potentization' and other homeopathic terms.

Each of the laws and principles have been expressed in a simplified manner without omitting any of the essential content. A reading list is included on page 68 for those students wishing to explore the subject in more detail.

Whether your aim is to use your knowledge of homeopathy for first aid in the home, or you are hoping to continue your studies in order to practice professionally, an understanding of the basic principles of its philosophy is essential. These principles have remained virtually unchanged since the system was developed 200 years ago.

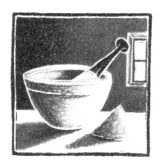

What is homeopathy?

Homeopathy is a system of medicine which respects the fact that every person is a unique individual. This 'holistic' approach treats the whole person, not just the disease. It is deep acting and addresses every level of the patient's being - physical, mental, emotional and spiritual.

 What does 'homeopathy' mean?

The word 'homeopathy' comes from the ancient Greek language and means "similar suffering". Breaking the word down, *homios* means **like** and *pathos* means **suffering**, and has nothing to do with the Latin word *homo* - **man**. In contrast, conventional medicine, which is based on the principle of opposites, was termed 'allopathy' by Hahnemann (see page 19), from the Greek *allos* - **other**.

 What is a homeopathic remedy?

The difference between a remedy that has been homeopathically prepared and the original substance it was prepared from is in the process of dilution and potentization (as explained on page 35) which renders the substance harmless while retaining its beneficial properties.

Over the past 200 or so years information on the origins, medicinal properties and clinical use of these substances has been recorded in books called **Materia Medica**. New remedies are continually being added as records become available.

Remedies are made from substances as far ranging as **Sepia**, (cuttlefish) from the animal kingdom; **Bellis Perennis**, (common daisy), from the vegetable world and from the sphere of minerals, volcanic **Sulphur**.

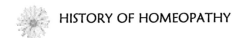

The use of homeopathy goes back much further than many people realise. Hieroglyphics provide us with evidence from ancient Egypt that a form of homeopathy was in use even then. And over 3,000 years ago, Hindu writings taught homeopathy as a theory as well as a means of treatment.

Over the next few centuries the seeds of homeopathic thought lay dormant and were largely forgotten, until in the 5th Century BC. **Hippocrates**, a prominent Greek physician, developed the theory, practice and study of medicine into an art and a science. **Hippocrates** recognised that there were two main ways of treating disease and wrote that healing could be accomplished by:

1   the use of **contraries**, or

2   the use of **similars** (homeopathy).

The first of these - using **contraries**, or allopathic medicine - uses a medicament to oppose or counteract the symptoms of disease, for example, a laxative to ease constipation.

The second - treating 'like with like' (or '**similars**') - stimulates the natural healing force in the body by administering a substance, or remedy, which mimics (copies) the signs and symptoms of the illness (see below). This use of **similars** is the basis of homeopathy and was another step towards its current practice. See page 29.

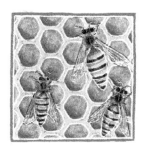

Law of Similars.
A sting from the honey bee can cause inflammation, redness and itching. A remedy made from the same substance will speedily relieve these symptoms even though the cause may not have been a bee sting.

Hippocrates was the first to appreciate the significance of hygiene, environmental factors, diet and a healthy way of life, believing that the body was able to heal itself.

Hippocrates is quoted as stating:

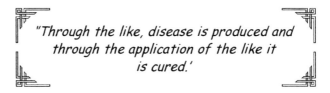

"Through the like, disease is produced and through the application of the like it is cured.'

The Hippocratic way of medicine was followed throughout the ancient world until, with the growth of Christianity, the approach to medicine in the West began to change.

In the 2nd century AD, **Galen**, a famous physician and theorist of his day, whilst accepting the importance of **Hippocrates'** work, developed his own ideas. He believed in using contraries to force out disease with the use of numerous drugs.

Galen systematically set about rationalising medical thought, emphasizing the importance of treatment by opposites while treatment by the use of similars became neglected and forgotten. His authoritarian ideas dominated medical science for centuries and physicians found any departure from his dogmatic theories very difficult.

An example of this influence is evident even in relatively modern times when **Harvey**, who discovered the circulation of blood in the body, was ridiculed because it was not in accordance with **Galen's** theories.

Galen's idea of treatment by opposites dominates medical thinking from that day to this.

The next significant development towards homeopathy came from a prominent 16th Century philosopher and physician, **Paracelsus**. His reputation as 'the Father of Chemistry' came about when he updated the theory of 'alchemy' and the search for the elixir of life.

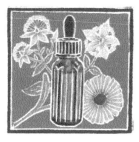 His ideas were based on pharmacological study and observation of plants, animals and minerals, applying his findings to the treatment of illness. **Paracelsus**, too, came to believe in 'like cures like', or that the poison causing a disease should become its cure.

He went on to prove this by curing a village of the plague with medicine made from minute amounts of the villagers' own excreta. Once again, his observations were ahead of their time and it was not until two hundred years later that a German doctor, **Samuel Hahnemann**, continued and developed this theme.

The Father of Homeopathy

Christian Friedrich Samuel **Hahnemann** was born in Meissen, East Germany in 1755 into a family of five children. His family were poor and held strong Protestant beliefs and high principles. His father taught him to question everything and would set him problems to solve and lock him in his room to think them through. He would not be allowed out until he had found the solution.

Samuel was such a bright child that his teachers waived his fees in order to allow him to continue his education. He was teaching Greek to his fellow students at the age of 12, and by 20, was fluent in 8 languages. Around this time, he enrolled at the University of Leipzig, where he studied medicine and chemistry qualifying as a doctor in 1779. As with modern day students, whilst at the University Hahnemann had had to find work to support himself, and this he did by doing translation work for scientific publishers.

Marrying young, Hahnemann became frustrated at his inability to adequately treat his own children's ailments due to the poor choice of medicine available. In fact, during his nine years of general practice, he became increasingly disillusioned by the cruel and ineffective treatments of the day. These included giving crude doses of dangerous substances such as mercury, arsenic and opium and large doses of purgatives.

Blood-letting and leeching was thought to relieve high blood pressure by allowing poisons to escape from the body, and was common practice. Operations were seldom accompanied by any form of antiseptic and cross-infections leading to fatalities were common. These barbaric practices caused dreadful suffering to patients who were already weakened and no longer had the energy to fight their illness.

Around this time, medical researchers were experimenting with extracting the active ingredients from plants and this undoubtedly attracted Hahnemann's attention.

Fortunately for the future of homeopathy, Hahnemann decided to give up his practice and returned to his translation work to support his wife and growing family in order to pursue his chemical and botanical studies.

> "...I renounced the practice of medicine, that I
> might no longer incur the risk of doing injury, and I
> engaged exclusively on chemistry and in literary
> occupations...."

In 1790 whilst translating 'A Treatise on Materia Medica' by Dr William Cullen, his interest was aroused by an item on quinine, a substance extracted from Peruvian Bark, otherwise known as China Officianalis.

Dr Cullen found quinine to be a most effective remedy for the relief of malaria. He felt the disease was cured by the astringent or bitter qualities of the material.

However, Hahnemann was aware that there were many plant products even more bitter than quinine and he knew that they were ineffective against malaria. Not satisfied with Dr Cullen's theory, Hahnemann started to experiment on himself. He would take 'twice a day, four drachms' of China, and to his surprise he began to exhibit the symptoms of malaria, the very disease that quinine was supposed to cure.

He deduced from this important discovery, that by observing the symptoms a substance produced when taken by a healthy person, he could discover what the healing properties of that substance were. This method he called 'Proving' and it is one of the basic principles of present day homeopathy. See page 31.

A notable example of Hahnemann's work describes his observation of an artist friend who had become physically weakened and unusually indifferent to his loved ones. Watching his friend at work, Hahnemann noticed the artist repeatedly sucking the tip of his paint brush which was coated in sepia ink, a substance made from the juice of the cuttlefish. After making a  homeopathic remedy from the ink, he prescribed it for his friend whose condition rapidly improved.

Hahnemann devoted himself to the research of the medicinal application of a variety of substances, constantly updating his theories, publishing in 1810 and 1811 his famous works entitled 'Organon of Rational Medicine' and 'Materia Medica'.

One of Hahnemann's well-documented early successes was after the Battle of Leipzig in 1813 when, during an epidemic of typhoid, he treated 180 patients with homeopathic remedies and only one died. Those given conventional medicine suffered far greater fatalities.

Unfortunately, Hahnemann was becoming increasingly unpopular with apothecaries and physicians because, not only was he preparing his own remedies, the province of the apothecaries, but also his theories challenged the practices of the physicians!

1820 heralded further difficult years for Hahnemann when the apothecaries persuaded the government to grant an injunction against him, preventing him from dispensing his own remedies.

During this time he enjoyed the support of Prince Karl Schwarzenberg of Austria whose health was improving under his ministrations. Prince Karl wrote to King Friedrich of Austria urging him to lift the ban on Hahnemann, but unfortunately the Prince died of a stroke and Hahnemann was unfairly blamed. His work was ridiculed and burnt in public.

Hahnemann, by now 65 years old, was invited by Grand Duke Ferdinand to live in Cothen in East Germany where he remained for the next 14 years, working as a court physician but never abandoning the development of his theories on homeopathy.

Following the death of his first wife when he was 79, Hahnemann met and married a young French woman, Melanie d'Hervilly, who had travelled from Paris to consult Hahnemann professionally. She helped her husband with his now successful practice, run on a 'no-cure-no-fee' system and they remained very happy together until his death on 2 July 1843 at the age of 88.

Samuel Hahnemann
1755-1843

A
Different
Approach
to
Health

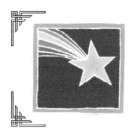

A Different
Approach
to Health

As a holistic therapy, homeopathy recognises that symptoms of illness are expressions of disharmony, or dis-ease, within the whole person and that it is the person and not the illness that needs treatment. When a person is unwell or under stress, their body attempts to restore balance, a process in which symptoms are displayed, e.g. headaches, feeling sick, painful joints etc. Viewed in this way, symptoms can be seen as the external effects of the internal fight to get well.

Hahnemann advocated the use of substances which work with the body, encouraging it to throw off the symptoms of illness by stimulating its own natural healing energy. Because these symptoms, to a homeopath, are a positive sign that the body's own natural defence mechanism is at work, they are noted and prescribed upon, according to the individual, to effect a cure.

For example, a sore throat may be accompanied by a **fever**. which is actually a healthy response to bacterial or viral invasion. The rise in temperature is a by-product of the increased number of white blood cells produced to combat the infection. These cells become more active, producing a body protein called interferon which burns off the invading agent preventing an increase in its growth.   The allopathic approach suppresses these characteristic symptoms with anti-inflammatory drugs such as aspirin, or antibiotics.

In contrast, the homeopathic approach is to offer support through the various stages enabling the illness to clear up more quickly and with the minimum amount of complication. Because homeopathy attempts to match an individual's symptom picture with the appropriate remedy (Law of Similars, see page 29), it is of little relevance whether the infection is of bacterial or viral origin.

Similarly, if the catarrhal discharge of the **common cold** is suppressed with nasal sprays or decongestants, further problems may occur. Catarrh is simply toxic waste containing dead white blood cells, viruses, bacteria and mucous which the body needs to be rid of. The suppression of this function is likely to drive the illness deeper, where it could have a more serious impact on the person's health.

Conventional medicine sees symptoms as problems that have to be suppressed or eradicated. These important signals may be prescribed upon for a long time or even on a permanent basis and the unwanted side-effects of continued drug use often result in chronic ill-health.

Another problem is the increasing amount of specialisation which singles out individual organs such the brain, heart, liver or kidneys for specific treatment, isolating them from the synchronised working of the body as a whole. Treatment focusing on specific organs can result in a patient being prescribed different tablets for different disorders all at the same time and incompatibilities often arise. Unfortunately, modern science regards 'good health' as the absence of symptoms rather than the positive acquiring of a healthy and well-regulated body.

The homeopathic approach encourages the body to find its own balance and harmony by combining natural methods and medicines with the body's innate wisdom, thus promoting self-healing.

'The highest ideal of cure is rapid, gentle, and permanent restoration of the health, or removal of the disease in its whole extent in the shortest, most reliable and most harmless way, on easily comprehensible principles'.

Samuel Hahnemann.   1810.

The
Principles
of
Homeopathy

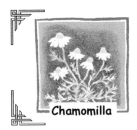

Chamomilla

The
Law of Similars

One of the most important principles of homeopathy is the concept of 'like cures like', (*similia similibus curentur*) otherwise known as the Law of Similars. This means that an agent or substance that can harm or cause disease can also cure.

For instance, coffee is a substance which stimulates the nervous system and can keep you awake, therefore causing sleeping difficulties.

The way of similars is to give a minute dose of *coffea*, made from coffee which, because it matches the symptom picture of sleeplessness, stimulates the inbuilt capacity of the body to heal itself, soothing the nerves and resulting in natural sleep.

Imagine you have a minor cut on your hand from a piece of broken glass. As soon as a message reaches your brain that the skin has been injured, healing forces are mobilised, triggering a response to the need to repair the damage.

A homeopathic remedy has the power to stimulate this same response by helping your body to recognise what it has to do to restore itself.

It is this basic idea that Hahnemann took and developed into a full therapeutic system using 'similars' to treat illness.

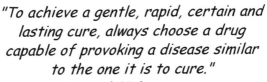

"To achieve a gentle, rapid, certain and lasting cure, always choose a drug capable of provoking a disease similar to the one it is to cure."
Samuel Hahnemann

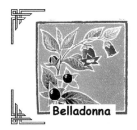
Belladonna

Provings

By observing the symptoms a substance produced when taken by a healthy person, Hahnemann realised he had discovered what the healing properties of that substance were.

Following his own provings of Peruvian Bark, or China (as discussed in the History of Homeopathy - see also overleaf), he went on to give controlled doses of the substance to friends and family in order to verify his findings.

They were asked to take daily doses over a period of time and record the effects. These volunteers, who were in good health, were instructed to observe closely and record in great detail any symptoms, emotional or physical, that affected them. They were not allowed to compare notes, and strict dietary conditions were imposed upon them. These included the avoidance of stimulants such as alcohol, tea and coffee, to avoid confusing the results.

Once this procedure became established, and the results meticulously recorded, Hahnemann began to research other medicinal, and sometimes poisonous, substances such as arsenic and belladonna in the same way. The symptoms which occurred most frequently became known as 'keynotes' and the combination of symptoms from the substances tested made up a therapeutic remedy picture for each.

Hahnemann also researched accounts of poisonings and drug use throughout the centuries in medical libraries. This information was collated and added to his provings, combining to form the Materia Medica as we know it today.

'As an experiment, I took about 4 drachms of good quality China twice daily for a number of days. First my feet, fingertips etc. grew cold and I became languid and drowsy. Then I developed palpitations, my pulse grew hard and rapid, intolerable anxiety, tremor (but no shivering) and enervation in all limbs. Then a pulse was beating in my head, redness of cheeks, thirst - in short all the symptoms familiar to me as belonging to intermittent fever made their appearance one after the other, though there were no actual attacks of chills and fever. In short, the highly characteristic symptoms of intermittent fever I am familiar with - dullness of the senses, a kind of stiffness in all joints, and above all the unpleasant sensation of numbness which seemed to be located in the periosteum of all the bones in my body - all made their appearance. The paroxysms always lasted for 2 or 3 hours, recurring only when I repeated the dose. I stopped taking the drug and I was well again.'

Quotation taken from
Samuel Hahnemann's proving
of Peruvian Bark

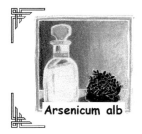

The Law
of the
Minimum Dose

Arsenicum alb

While Hahnemann could see that many medicines in use at that time had valuable properties, he became frustrated as many were poisonous or had unpleasant side effects. These medicines were so powerful that they could just as easily kill as cure.

He experimented with more and more **dilution** of the substances, hoping to retain the beneficial properties while losing the harmful ones, but got to a point where they became altogether ineffective. His aim was to be able to administer the smallest dose possible to effect a cure, but on reaching this impasse, legend has it that

instead of stirring his mixture as usual, Hahnemann resorted to striking a small bottle of the medicinal substance repeatedly on a leather bound Bible.

To his surprise, he discovered that not only had the medicinal properties been retained but also strength and energy had been released, making the remedy more potent thus enhancing the remedial effect. This action Hahnemann later termed "**succussion**" and repeated it after each stage of dilution until he reached the strength required.

Hahnemann called the combined process of dilution and succussion '**dynamization**' - in other words, the point at which a crude substance somehow makes the transition into energetic or dynamic medicine.

By continuing to test other substances, which in their natural form are completely inert, such as calcium and silica, Hahnemann found these also yielded curative effects when subjected to this process.

This major breakthrough resulted in Hahnemann's potentised medicines which he called Remedies.

Armed with this new idea Hahnemann proceeded to dynamize more and more substances, rendering each of them harmless but effective. These included popular medicaments of the day such as Opium, Arsenic and Mercury. He was thus able to administer the **minimum dose** which was needed to effect the desired curative reponse.

The Arndt-Schultz Law

Hahnemann's experiments, performed some two hundred years ago, reflect a present day law of chemistry - the Arndt-Schultz Law. This Law decrees that small stimuli encourage living systems, medium stimuli impede them and strong stimuli tend to stop or destroy them altogether.

"All things are poison, it is the dosage that makes a thing not poison."
Paracelsus

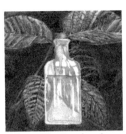

Rhus Toxicodendron

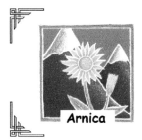

Arnica

Potentization

Hahnemann invented a potency scale for his remedies identifying each stage of dilution. The number you may see associated with a homeopathic remedy, such as Arnica 30c, indicates the number of times the substance has passed through the dilution and succussion process, thus indicating its strength.

The 'c' shown after the number stands for 'centesimal' which is Latin for 100. This is because one drop of the original substance is mixed with 99 parts of a water/alcohol solution, making one hundred drops and then succussed to make the 1c potency. From this new mixture, one drop is taken and added to 99 parts of the water/alcohol solution, and again succussed thus creating a 2c. When this process has been followed thirty times, you have a remedy in the 30c potency.

Hahnemann's research established that the more times this potentization (or dynamization) process was repeated, the more powerful the medicine became.

This answers the question of why Arnica 30c is a more powerful dose than Arnica 6c in spite of the fact that is is further away from the original substance. It is the dynamic action of dilution and succussion that energises the substance.

You can see that the **Law of Similars** was of no practical use until the related **Law of the Minimum Dose** and the principle of **Potentization** were developed.

In 1839 **Hahnemann** wrote:

'Homeopathic dynamizations genuinely bring to life the medicinal properties which lie hidden in natural solids when these are in the crude state.'

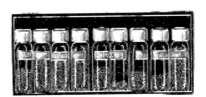

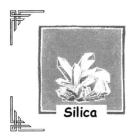

Silica

The
Vital Force

As **Hahnemann** continued to refine his ideas, he concluded that remedies appeared to affect a part of the person that was non-material. This part he called the **'vital force'** - the spirit that motivates the mind and uses the body for its physical expression. When this 'vital force' is upset by an external factor, such as stress or an injury, it attempts to redress the balance in the body and this is when symptoms of illness may appear.

The idea of the presence of an invisible, yet tangible 'vital force' is an ancient one. The *'Prana'* of the Hindus, or the Chinese, *'Chi'*, that elusive quality which departs at death, is the principle which animates spirit, soul and energy.

Another way of viewing the vital force is to see it as an organising intelligence that runs all the different control systems of the body, such as the immune system, autonomic nervous system, the hormonal system etc. and is capable of stimulating the body's own healing response when necessary.

This innate protective device provides 'homeostasis' (the maintenance of a stable system), adjusting and balancing us every second of our lives, e.g. shivering when cold, sleeping when tired, or producing a fever to burn off infection.

Conventional medicine suppresses the vital force and weakens the defence mechanism. Homeopathic treatment stimulates the vital force, strengthening the defence mechanism and the patient will tell you that he feels 'better in himself', a sure sign of healing at work.

"In the healthy condition of man, the spiritual vital force (autocracy), the dynamism that animates the material body (organism), rules with unbounded sway, and retains all the parts of the organism in admirable, harmonious, vital operation, as regards both sensations and function, so that our indwelling, reason-gifted mind can freely employ this living, healthy instrument for the higher purposes of our existence."

Samuel Hahnemann - The Organon.

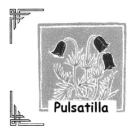
Pulsatilla

Totality
of Symptoms

After a detailed consultation with the patient, (which may last an hour or more), the aim of the homeopath is to select a remedy which most closely matches the **totality of symptoms** and not just individual signs and symptoms. This remedy should cover all aspects of the problem, mental, emotional and physical. This demonstrates the holistic approach to disease practised in homeopathy.

Signs of illness are unique to each person. My headache will be different to your headache. Your child's earache will vary from my child's because one of the symptoms displayed may be that one is thirsty, indicating Sulphur. The other refuses drinks and Pulsatilla could be the remedy of choice. Choosing the most suitable remedy will depend on the totality of the symptoms exhibited by the individual.

Although you should always have this principle in the back of your mind, it is not always possible to adhere to for the purposes of First Aid. Prompt action is needed and therefore your leading symptoms are likely to be physical and obvious. There is no time to take a detailed medical history when the casualty is bleeding profusely or has just fallen off a ladder! However, in the case of severe shock, when deciding between Arnica or Aconite, you will need to consider not only the physical, but also the mental or emotional state of the patient.

"A single symptom is no more the whole disease than a single foot is the whole man".

Samuel Hahnemann

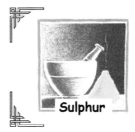
Sulphur

Hering's Law of the Direction of Cure

A major contribution to homeopathy was made by the 19th century American homeopath, **Constantine Hering**. As a university medical student, he was asked by his tutors to investigate Hahnemann's work with a view to discrediting it. Far from doing this, it captured his interest and he became a convert to homeopathy.

During the course of his studies, he observed that the progress of cure in constitutional treatment always appeared to take the same course, i.e.

- · from the inside to the outside
- · from the top to the bottom
- · from the most important organs to less important organs
- · symptoms return in the reverse order of their appearance.

This Law is recognised in various forms by all the major medical systems of the world except conventional western medicine. Then, as now, homeopaths use this Law to monitor their cases and to check that cure is progressing correctly.

An example of Hering's Law is of a child who developed eczema which 'disappeared' with the use of steroid creams. The same child later suffered from hayfever, for which antihistamines were prescribed. Finally, he began to experience asthma attacks for which more steroids were given.

In orthodox medicine, these events would not have been connected and it would have been assumed that each had been 'cured'. But according to **Hering's Law of the Direction of Cure,** the child's health could have been seen to be gradually deteriorating. The focus of the illness started on his skin (irritating and uncomfortable) and ended in the respiratory organs (life-threatening). **Suppression** of the eczema drove the disease deeper into his system, thus beginning the journey into chronic ill-health.

After eventually consulting a homeopath, his treatment began with gentle removal of the asthma symptoms. The next stage in this particular case was the reappearance of hayfever, (inner to outer and major to minor organs).

Again regular use of remedies was employed until the symptoms subsided and a rash appeared on his skin - eczema, (inside to outside). Continued prescribing by the use of similars for the eczema symptoms encouraged the rash to travel down his body until ultimately it cleared completely (top to bottom).

Proving the Law of the Direction of Cure, the symptoms had returned in the reverse order of their appearance.

Susceptibility and Constitution

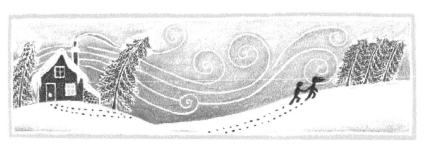

Susceptibility is the degree to which a person is vulnerable to outside influences. These influences can be many and varied and combine to produce the fundamental structure of that person, known as their basic **constitution**.

The biggest of these influences is likely to be what has been inherited through the family line in terms of strengths (e.g. absence of serious illness); and weaknesses (e.g. T.B., heart disease, cancer, syphilis, nervous disposition, etc). See **Miasms**, page 45.

Other factors include how this genetic inheritance has been modified by the individual's environment (i.e. all the things that have happened since conception and birth up to and including current life style).

*"**Susceptibility** is merely the name for a state that underlies all possible sickness and all possible cure".*
James Tyler Kent

All these combined experiences, whether genetic or acquired, determine whether a person is particularly healthy or has a tendency towards certain diseases. These weaknesses may manifest in specific organs, allergic conditions or in neurological stress, such as depression or mental illness.

We all have acquaintances who burn the candle at both ends, smoking and drinking as if there was no tomorrow and who boast about never ever having a cold! These individuals are not just 'lucky', but have been born of healthy parents from whom they have inherited their strong **constitution**. If they are not careful about the 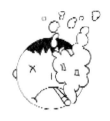 way they lead their lives, they are in danger of losing their inherited good health.

A person with a strong **constitution** is more likely to maintain better health than someone with a weak **constitution**, who will have an increased **susceptibility** to illness. This explains why not everyone in the office catches 'flu at the same time or why one child in the family contracts chickenpox but her siblings do not.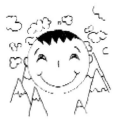

No two people react to a disease in the same way, as we each have our own highly individual way of expressing symptoms, influenced by our genetic inheritance. Likewise, each person copes differently with the problems and stresses of everyday life in an attempt to maintain inner balance. This combination of **susceptibility** and **constitutional** strength is an essential factor in **constitutional** prescribing by a homeopath.

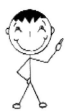 Those who do not abuse their health and take an active role in maintaining a sensible lifestyle, are far more likely to pass on the gift of **constitutional** health and well-being to successive generations.

> *"Ask not what kind of illness the patient has, ask what kind of patient has the illness."*
> **Sir William Osler**

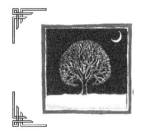

Miasms
an
introduction

Hahnemann formulated his theory of **miasms** when he observed that some patients failed to respond to their constitutional remedy, and others relapsed a short time after improvement.

After considerable clinical experience, he recognised the presence of certain disease patterns in the patient's personal history. He believed that this created a block to their constitutional health. These disease patterns were usually inherited, and he called them **miasms**.

Hahnemann described the three basic miasms as:

· **Psora** (suppressed skin itch)
· **Syphilis** (suppressed syphilis)
· **Sycosis** (suppressed gonorrhoea)

He felt that the variety of symptoms displayed in chronic disease arose from the continued passage of these infections through countless generations, predisposing a person to a particular range of health problems.

This theory attracted a great deal of scepticism and ridicule in his lifetime, an attitude which persisted until fairly recently. It is now known that the DNA of certain viruses can incorporate itself into the genes, thus passing to future generations. Subsequently, extra layers or 'blocks', such as **Tuberculosis** and **Cancer**, have since contributed to the miasmatic inheritance of the human condition.

Therefore, Hahnemann's perception that disease is due to a combination of inherited and environmental factors has turned out to be not only a very sound theory, but also provides the key to the homeopathic treatment of chronic illness.

The theory of **miasms** is fascinating but complex, therefore further study is recommended to enable the student to assimilate these ideas (see Reading List, page 68).

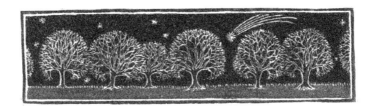

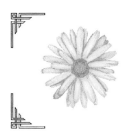

The
Single Remedy

The prescribing of a single remedy at the end of a homeopathic consultation is a basic principle of classical homeopathy. The idea behind it is that once the chosen remedy has initiated a healing response it should be allowed to run its course. A particularly well selected remedy is able to instigate a healing response that can continue for a long time, maybe months or even years.

Because each person responds differently to the remedy they have been given, the homeopath uses their symptom picture as a guide to how often to repeat the remedy.

Classical homeopaths believe that as all the remedies in the Materia Medica were proved separately, combining remedies makes it impossible to tell accurately which remedy has caused the beneficial reaction. This applies to **constitutional** treatment in particular.

'...when remedies cure they do so only through their ability to alter human health by causing characteristic symptoms...'

Samuel Hahnemann

Acute
and
Chronic
Prescribing

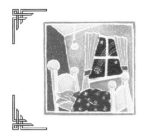

Acute
Illness

An **acute** illness comes on quickly and usually goes away sooner or later by itself. There are three stages to an **acute** illness:

- · the **incubation period**, when symptoms are rarely apparent
- · the **acute phase**, where the symptoms become visible
- · the **convalescent stage**, as the patient starts to recover.

Take the example of chickenpox, which has an **incubation period** of 7-21 days. The **acute phase** follows, with fever or general malaise, and the eruption of an irritating rash which develops into watery blisters.

The blisters burst and crust over to form scabs, signalling the **convalescent stage**, or in other words, return to health.

Note: *Chickenpox is infectious from the beginning of the incubation period until the last spot has scabbed over.*

Hahnemann's view was that in an **acute** illness, the **vital force** of the patient was either able to overcome the illness or alternatively the illness would rapidly overcome the **vital force**. In other words the person would either get better or die!

A person who has general good health and a strong vitality (**vital force**) will quickly be able to throw off an **acute** complaint. The symptoms experienced are signs of the body's attempt to rebalance itself and return to health.

This is a natural response of the immune system and is the point at which a well chosen remedy can aid the process considerably. Homeopathic remedies work with the body by stimulating its defence systems, thus speeding up the healing process.

Examples of **acute** illness include colds, flu, earaches, diarrhoea and vomiting, and childhood infectious illnesses. More serious, and potentially life-threatening **acute** problems such as meningitis or pneumonia, need urgent medical attention and fast prescribing by a qualified practitioner.

An **acute** illness that develops complications could turn into a **chronic** condition as detailed on the next page.

--ooOOoo--

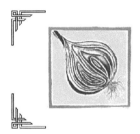

Chronic Conditions

Chronic complaints can come from either hereditary or environmental sources. The onset of this type of illness is insidious, resulting in deep-rooted problems for future generations. They can be of a serious or minor nature, developing gradually and continuing for a long time, usually accompanied by a general deterioration of health and worsening of symptoms.

It is also possible for a **chronic** illness to develop from an **acute** illness. For example, a bout of rheumatic fever (**acute**) can cause complications because of its effect on muscles, including the heart (**chronic**). Rheumatic fever may also affect the joints, leaving the patient with rheumatic pains (**chronic**).

Such complications are unlikely to clear up by themselves because they cannot be eradicated by the **vital force** alone. However regular homeopathic treatment by a qualified practitioner can alleviate symptoms, halt the progress of the disease and by stimulating the **vital force**, can result in a gentle and effective return to health.

The treatment of **chronic** illness has been compared to peeling an onion composed of many layers. Each layer represents an illness, accident or trauma experienced by the individual. Homeopathic treatment works by removing each layer in turn, including the inherited disease patterns of our forebears, eventually restoring health and vitality.

Some examples of serious chronic illness include asthma, arthritis, rheumatism, depression, heart disease, cancer and skin problems such as eczema and psoriasis.

Dozens of less serious conditions are actually minor chronic problems. Examples include dandruff, persistent catarrh, warts or haemorrhoids, and pre-menstrual syndrome.

All of these problems can be greatly relieved and often cured by homeopathic remedies which address the underlying cause of the problem.

--ooOOoo--

How
to Use
Remedies

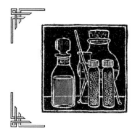

How to Use Remedies

Remedies are obtainable from most large chemists or health food shops. They are usually available in 6x, 6c and 30c potencies which are most appropriate for general use. Specialist homeopathic pharmacies will supply stronger doses if required direct from their shop or by telephone order.

The Remedy

Homeopathic medicines are supplied in various forms:

Sucrose based:

· pillules (pills)
· granules (the size of poppy seeds)

Lactose based:

· trituration tablets (often as Tissue Salts *). Useful for babies.
· individually wrapped powders

Combined sucrose and lactose:

· hard tablets.

All homeopathic remedies can be made up in liquid form and supplied in a dropper bottle.

Because of the way they are prepared, no toxic substances are involved (see Principles of Philosophy - potentization), therefore there can be no danger from overdosing or addiction. Homeopathic remedies are completely safe for anyone to use, including pregnant mums, newborn babies, elderly people and also animals.

Potency

Homeopathic remedies come in a variety of strengths which are known as potencies. When first embarking on the use of remedies the safest potencies for the home prescriber are the 6x (commonly used for tissue salts*), 6c, or 30c.

You will find remedies in the 6c or 30c potency most appropriate for home prescribing. They are easily obtainable from pharmacies and health food shops. High (or stronger) potencies e.g. 200c, need less frequent repetition to achieve the desired result and should always be discussed with a qualified practitioner before prescribing.

In an emergency or first aid situation, if all you have is a low potency, do not hold back from using it as it may just need more frequent repetition than a higher one. The choice of remedy which most closely matches the symptoms is more important than the potency.

---

* Tissue Salts (Biochemic therapeutic system of twelve tissue remedies introduced by Dr Wilhelm Schussler) - a system of replacing a mineral salt deficiency in the body with its potentised homeopathic form (e.g. Kali Sulphuricum - potassium sulphate; Natrum Muriaticum - sodium chloride). Common potency used is a 6x.

Taking the Remedy

Because of the subtle nature of homeopathic remedies, it is important to handle them as little as possible to avoid contamination. Therefore tip one pill into the lid of the bottle (returning extras until only one remains), then transfer it straight into the mouth of the patient if possible, or on to a sterilised spoon (especially useful for babies or infirm people). Replace the lid on the bottle quickly. If the pills are in a packet, follow the same procedure.

The pill should be dissolved under the tongue, where it is readily absorbed by the mucous membranes of the mouth.   If necessary, pills and tablets can be crushed or dissolved in water and sipped, but should never be washed down with a drink.

Nothing should be put in your mouth for twenty minutes before or after taking the remedy in order to give it the best chance of working. This includes food, drink, chewing gum, toothpaste, sweets and cigarettes.

Sometimes leaving this time gap can be difficult, especially in emergency situations, or when administering to babies or small children. In this case give the remedy anyway and repeat it a few minutes later to ensure that any food residue, etc. has not affected the action of the remedy.

In emergencies, administer the remedy as above while waiting for the medical services to arrive.

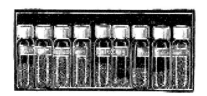

Dosage

In *minor* complaints, e.g. a bruise or a chill, repeat the **6c** dosage *three to six times in 24 hours*.

For a *more serious* complaint with unpleasant symptoms which are not necessarily accompanied with great pain, e.g. sickness or diarrhoea, repeat the **30c** dosage every *one to two hours* until improvement, then **STOP** and evaluate the action of the remedy, see below.

A *very serious* complaint would include symptoms needing immediate attention, often accompanied by a lot of pain: e.g. a severe injury or burn. Repeat the **30c** dosage every *five to thirty minutes*, as needed, slowing down the frequency to match the rate of recovery.

Evaluate the effect of the remedy.

The Law of the Minimum Dose says we must only use as little of a medicine as possible to stimulate the body's own healing mechanism. When you see a definite change as a result of giving the remedy, reduce the frequency of the dosage until a marked improvement is noted. Then **STOP**. If the same symptoms return, repeat the dose.

If there has been no marked improvement after 3-4 doses, double-check the symptoms as you may have selected the wrong remedy. You may need to change your prescription if the original symptoms have improved but new ones appear, or if the remedy picture has changed - which is frequently the case in emergency situations.

The golden rule is to stop the remedy on improvement allowing your body to continue the healing process without further interference.

Examples

Sometimes combinations of remedies are used therapeutically, especially in first aid or acute situations. For example, it would be very difficult to adequately treat a severely shocked burns casualty with only one remedy. In this instance a dose of **Arnica 30c** (you would be unlikely to have a higher dose in a standard first aid kit) would allow the shock element to be released, after which repeated doses of the appropriate burns remedy can be given - **two-hourly** until improvement in the **6c** or **30c** potency.

Similarly, a bout of influenza passes through different stages. It could be that as the symptoms change, different remedies will be needed to cover each phase of the illness. Giving the appropriate remedy at **two-hourly** intervals in the **30c** potency and changing it as the symptoms alter, speeds the rate of recovery, lessens discomfort and avoids unpleasant complications.

Antidoting

It is advisable to avoid certain things that are known to upset the curative response or even antidote the remedy outright, as follows:

Coffee	includes decaffeinated: coffee flavoured sweets and cakes.

Teas	China, Indian, fruit and herb teas are fine in moderation but avoid chamomile and peppermint.

Peppermint	includes tea, sweets, chocolate, chewing gum and toothpaste and body lotions.

Strong Substances	aromatherapy oils, <u>tea-tree oil</u> products, camphor, Olbas oil, Karvol, Deep Heat, Vicks, etc.

Menthol/ Eucalyptus	Vicks, Karvol, cough mixture, throat lozenges, vaporisers, aromatherapy oils and burners.

Drugs	Cannabis is a proven antidote.

X-rays and Radio Waves	keep remedies away from mobile phones, microwave ovens, electrical appliances and avoid taking through X-ray machines in airports.

Adrenalin	before visiting the dentist, ask your homeopath for advice about the components of the injection.

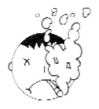 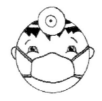

Coffee alternatives include Caro, Bambu, Dandelion Coffee, No-Caf. Despite initial resistance, you'll be surprised how easy it is to stop drinking coffee altogether!

Hollytrees and Kingfisher produce non-mint and non-fluoride toothpastes in lemon, orange and fennel flavours. Explore your local healthfood shop or chemist for these and other brands.

Storage

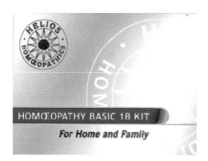

HOMŒOPATHY BASIC 18 KIT

For Home and Family

Remedies need careful handling and storage to preserve their quality and prevent them from becoming inert as a result of contamination. Store in a cool dark place and keep away from heat, strong light, odours and electrical appliances e.g. TVs, mobile phones, microwaves, and computers.

When flying, keep your remedies in a lead-lined camera case to avoid radiation which might affect their efficiency.

Keep remedies in the container in which you receive them and never transfer them to any other packet or bottle, in order to avoid cross-contamination. If you drop a pill, never return it to the container as replacing it could risk spoiling the remainder.

All medication should be kept out of the reach of children. If your child accidentally 'eats' a bottle of remedies, don't panic! Because there are no toxic side effects, no harm can be done.

Apart from High Street Chemists and health food shops, homeopathic pharmacies stock a comprehensive range of remedies, creams and tinctures, and relevant reading matter.

Remedy kits are also available nowadays and provide you with a convenient range of remedies for every day use. These are available by mail order. For further information, telephone:

HealthWorks
01622 842311

Useful Addresses

For homeopathic stationery and remedy kits
HealthWorks
20 Ashford Drive
Kingswood
Maidstone
Kent ME17 3PB
Tel: 01622 842311
www.healthworksonline.co.uk

For mail order service for homeopathic supplies
Helios Homoeopathic Pharmacy
89-97 Camden Road
Tunbridge Wells
Kent TN1 2QR
Tel: 01892 537254/536393
www.helios.co.uk

For general information and register of qualified homeopaths
Homeopathic Medical Association
6 Livingstone Road
Gravesend
Kent DA12 5DZ
Tel: 01474 560336
www.the-hma.org

Send A5 SAE for regional list of registered homeopaths to
Society of Homeopaths
2 Artizan Road
Northampton
NN1 4HU
Tel: 01604 621400

GENERAL READING

For Newcomers to Homeopathy

Blackie, Margery G: *The Challenge of Homoeopathy.*

Hayfield, Robin: *Homoeopathy for Common Ailments,* Gaia Books, 1993

Osborne, Jean and Hool, Meryl: *Homeopathic Holiday Guide,* HealthWorks *2000*

Shepherd, Dorothy: *A Physician's Posy,* Health Science Press, 1969

Shepherd, Dorothy: *The Magic of the Minimum Dose,* Health Science Press, 1964

Shepherd, Dorothy: *More Magic of the Minimum Dose,* Health Science Press, 1974

Tyler, Margaret: *Homoeopathic Drug Pictures,* Health Science Press, 1952

Vithoulkas, George: *Homoeopathy, Medicine of the New Man,* Thorsons 1985

Watson, Ian: *Guide to Methodologies of Homoeopathy,* Cutting Edge Publications 1991

FURTHER READING

Coulter, Harris L: *Homoeopathic Science and Modern Medicine: the Physics of Healing with Microdoses,* North Atlantic Books 1987

Miles, Martin: *Homoeopathy and Human Evolution,* Winter Press, 1992

Vithoulkas, George: *The Science of Homoeopathy,* Thorsons *1986*

OTHER TITLES IN THE
SIMPLY HOMEOPATHY RANGE

THE HEALTHWORKS
HOMEOPATHIC HOLIDAY GUIDE

Bites and Stings, Sunburn, 'Traveller's Tummy',
Camping, Skiing, or Seaside holidays, Home or Flying Away -
the HealthWorks Holiday Guide provides you with advice on how to use a
basic range of remedies in the treatment of everyday problems
encountered on your holiday.

Simply presented in an easy to follow format with original colour
illustrations, the Holiday Guide is fully indexed and includes practical tips
for all your travel needs. Pack it in your bag!

ISBN 0-9538884-0-1

Sneezes and Wheezes
A BEGINNER'S GUIDE TO THE TREATMENT OF
COUGHS, COLDS, FEVERS AND FLU

Coughs and colds can strike at any time, sometimes just as a minor
inconvenience and at other times causing real problems when your life is
disrupted by the misery of incapacitating illness.

Sneezes and Wheezes has been written to acccompany the **Double Helix
Basic 36 Kit** and is presented in a simple, easy to read format, designed
to enable the reader to select the correct remedy for every situation
quickly and easily.

ISBN 0-9538884-2-8

HealthWorks